Crossfit Training

The Best Crossfit Workout Guide With Nutrition Tips For Maximum Results In Minimum Time

(Beginner's Workout Guide: The Complete Edition)

Coleman Daniel

TABLE OF CONTENT

Body Fat Measurement Techniques 1

Time-Restricted Eating Is Also Known As Intermittent Fasting 17

Be Aware Of Your Body. 37

The Risks Of Lacking Sleep 41

Crossfit Exercises 46

For Runners: Cross Training 52

Have You Considered The Fat Burning Cross Training Options Yet? 58

What Makes A Good Breakfast? 64

Cross-Training With A Paleo Diet 81

How Many Blocks Do You Need 89

Body Fat Measurement Techniques

Body fat is not measured by BMI. There are numerous methods for determining a body's amount of fat if you're interested in knowing your percentage of lean mass against fat mass. These techniques are known as body composition analysis. Some of the most popular measurements include:

Bioelectrical impedance: This popular technique for calculating body fat percentage determines total body weight, the percentage and amount of body fat, muscle mass, water, and even bone mass. While readings may be influenced by humidity level and other variables, they consistently provide very accurate results. Some body fat scales intended for home use employ this technique for measurement.

DEXA: Dual-energy x-ray absorptiometry This x-ray imager evaluates a person's bones (specifically their mineral density and bone loss) to calculate the likelihood of developing osteoporosis. But these DEXA devices have limitations, and the widely used technology cannot measure the bones in people who weigh 300 pounds or more or who are taller than 6 feet.

Measuring the thickness of the skin: This straightforward method is used by many experts to determine body composition.

Underwater wriggling: This process, also known as hydrometry or hydrostatic weighting, is complex and convoluted, which is why it is seldom used.

Although the body mass index might be a useful tool for certain people, it is just one figure that should always be taken into account within the context of other data. Speak with your healthcare practitioner about the best way to comprehend your BMI as part of a holistic strategy for long-term health.

Do you have concerns that you may be underweight? While many of the people around you may be concerned about the weight they are gaining, you may be concerned about the weight you are losing. What are the symptoms of being underweight, then? There are a few to which you should pay attention if you are really thin or losing weight rapidly.

What Is Underweight To You?

According to the Centers for Disease Control (CDC), if your body mass index (BMI) is lower than 18.5 you are considered underweight. You can calculate your BMI using a simple method. You must know your height and weight in order to enter them into the calculator:

Compare your results to the scores from the standardized body mass index.

18.5 or less: Unhealthy weight

18.5 to 24.9: A Normal Weight Range

Weighty between 25.0 and 29.9

Obese, BMI 30.0 or higher

Remember that the body mass index is not a diagnostic tool.1 If your BMI is below 18.5, you are not necessarily in danger as a result of your weight. BMI is only a classification system. It is used as a screening tool by your doctor and other health organizations to assess your weight and risk of contracting an illness. You may also measure your body fat percentage to determine your body size. Women should generally have body fat measurements of at least 10–13% to support basic bodily functions. Men need at least 2-5% for essential bodily processes. Following these suggestions may not be healthy for you. Government studies released in 2018 by the National

Center for Health Statistics estimate that just 1.5% of the population is underweight. About 1.2% of men and 1.8% of women are underweight, respectively. How can you tell for sure whether you are underweight then? Your health care provider may assess your weight and determine if you need to gain weight in order to improve your health.

The Symptoms of Being Underweight

You could notice various physical symptoms if you are underweight. However, several symptoms that are often related to thinness may have other origins. Do you have any arms, for instance, if you're underweight? Some people who are really skinny complain about having veiny arms. However, bodybuilders also have very little arm. Therefore, having veiny arms by themselves isn't usually a sign that you are too thin. Others complain about joints that seem overly big. Your bones and joints may seem more prominent if you are underweight and have very little muscle mass. However, having big bones or a more noticeable joint does not always indicate that you are severely underweight. Other signs of being underweight may include issues caused by malnutrition:

Drowsiness or weariness from anemia

Fragile bones

Hair loss

irregular menstruation cycles or issues becoming pregnant

Poor growth and development, particularly in underweight children

Weak immune system

What Should I Do if I Feel Unwell?

Your doctor is the best source of information if you believe you are underweight. Low body weight may have a variety of causes, and your health care provider can rule out conditions including cancer, thyroid disease, digestive problems, or medications. Additionally, there are behavioral causes of underweight such as stress or depression. But it's possible that you are underweight due to genetics, your level of activity, or simply because you don't eat enough.

How to Put On Weight While Retaining Health

If your doctor determines that you are underweight, he or she would likely advise that you gain weight by consuming nutritious foods.3 You may increase your caloric intake by focusing on nutritious sources of protein, grains, and healthy fats. A licensed dietitian may be able to help you develop meals and eating habits that will enable you to put on weight and develop a robust, healthy physique.

Types of CrossFit Diets That Exist Historically, CrossFit has supported a few dietary methods. Here is a brief introduction to three of the most well-known diets: the Zone diet, the Paleo diet, and the ketogenic diet.

Ketogenic Diet

This diet, often known as keto, encourages rapid weight loss.

CroFt and keto may be an extremely effective weight-loss combination.

One of the primary benefits only truly applies to CrossFitters who join with pre-existing health or metabolic issues. Keto may help lessen or reverse the consequences of things like type 2 diabetes and overall give you more energy, which is obviously beneficial for better performance in sports.

Going keto has several advantages, many of which may be put to use. directly to the effectiveness and general health of CrossFit.

Here are a few of the more significant ones:

• The keto diet is anti-inflammatory, meaning many of the foods one eats are filled with antioxidants and other bioactive compounds that reduce inflammation in your body's tissues. • Keto has been shown to help people lose a lot of weight. This aids in your recovery and protects you against many illnesses including diabetes and cancer.

• Some studies have shown that a high-fat, low-carb diet may significantly reduce or reverse poor metabolic health, which can lower your chance of developing a wide range of other diseases.

• The keto diet encourages a lot of protein and fiber, two nutrients that aid in muscle repair and foster satiety (essential for weight loss).

- Many keto dieters claim that after an initial adjustment period, they have more energy from living in ketosis than they had while consuming carbohydrates.

There are a few things to remember while following a ketogenic diet. First off, "eating keto" doesn't always guarantee you'll go into ketosis. It's a little more complicated than that. A calorie is still a calorie when everything is said and done. You won't achieve your objectives if you consume more calories than you should.

Cutting too many carbohydrates might reduce your performance. While some individuals report an improvement in performance, others discover that this diet is not right for them.

Furthermore, let's not confound being healthy with the ketogenic diet. Someone who follows a ketogenic diet and consumes a lot of healthy fats, vegetables, and lean protein will look and feel quite differently from someone who consumes bacon and cheeseburgers without buns.

Finally, it's crucial to comprehend how carbs function in the body. Every gram of carbohydrates you consume will result in the body holding onto 2-3 grams of water. You will lose a lot of water weight when you suddenly reduce your carbohydrate intake (thus the term "water cuts" among athletes who compete in weight classes). You could see a significant leap on the scale, but it doesn't indicate a change in your body composition; instead, it indicates that you're holding onto less water.

If you attempt the ketogenic diet, read some studies, comprehend how your body functions, and be realistic.

Diet Plan Zoning Intended to Reduce Inflammation and Balance The Zone Diet uses block accounting and a balanced macronutrient ratio (30/30/40) to ensure that you eat foods that keep you in a good "zone" for performance.

With the Zone diet, you're supposed to eat on a schedule, starting within an hour of waking up and continuing every three to four hours to maintain your energy level.

On the Zone diet, you can technically eat any meal, but whole foods are simpler to block out since they are simple to balance. Blocks are the Zone's equivalent of points, making this plan something akin to automated tracking. For a detailed explanation of the Zone diet, see this page.

One qualification to the Zone plan is that the recommended daily "blocks" for men and women are 11 and 14, respectively.

When you do the math, this recommendation is quite restrictive. when you could see weight loss when following this diet, it won't last for very long. Additionally, you could lack the energy necessary to effectively hit a Crooked Workout.

Fortunately, the strategy has a sound framework. You may tweak this plan for improved performance and health by adding more "blocks."

a Paleo diet

The Paleo Diet is the reigning champion of clean nutrition.

Since the sport's inception, CrossFit and the Paleo Diet have remained closely related. One factor in its popularity is the fact that it remarkably adheres to Greg Glamour's initial dietary advice from the 2002 CROFT Journal article "What Is Fitness?", which stated: "Eat meat and vegetables, nuts and seeds, some fruit, a little starch, and no sugar." Keep your consumption at levels that will support activity without increasing body fat. Gregory Glassman

Paleo encourages eating "food a caveman would eat." It has acted as a stimulus for weight loss in several CroFatters.

Be cautious, however. If your goal is to increase your lean body mass, you may need to include more starchy vegetables and increase your carbohydrate consumption from nutrient-rich sources if you exercise often or lead an active lifestyle. You may discover that our Paleo for Athletes book might help you strike a balance between healthy eating and competitiveness.

Time-Restricted Eating Is Also Known As Intermittent Fasting.

The most frequent definitions of intermittent fasting, usually referred to as time-restricted eating, include a 16-hour period each day during which no food is consumed and an 8-hour window during which all meals are taken.

Other protocols and time frames exist as well, but the 16 off, 8 on is the most common.

This means that if you have your first meal at, say, 10 am, you should eat your final meal before 6 pm. You are free to start your first meal at any time as long as the fast is at least 16 hours long. And the eating window was 8 hours.

Intermittent There are many well-researched benefits of dieting.

What occurs when you fast Insulin levels significantly decline and insulin activity rises.

Exogenously rising human growth hormones help in muscular growth and fat burning.

Fasting gives your body the chance to concentrate on waste removal and cell repair.

When you practice time-restricted eating, you consume fewer meals and perhaps less calories.

IF reduces oxidative stress and igniting.

IF has anti-aging effects.

Intermittent fasting is a simple practice that has many benefits. No meal change is necessary. I still advise you to eat healthily, however.

You may combine intermittent fasting with whatever diet you want to follow.

For the majority of individuals, intermittent fasting is safe.

Drawbacks of intermittent fasting

An excellent level of discipline is needed for intermittent fasting.

You could need to skip breakfast or dinner, or you might need to eat at a different time than your friends and family.

The Keto diet is a kind of ketogenesis.

The insanely popular By limiting (or eliminating) the consumption of carbohydrates and sugar, the ketogenic diet is a technique to replicate the benefits of fasting without actually fasting.

Follow this rule

75–80% fat

protein at 20–25%

5% carbohydrates, particularly from leafy green vegetables.

Popular keto meals

Bacon

Checker Thugh

Broccoli

Any lush green veggies, such as kale,

Heavy Cream

Butter

Pros The keto diet is safe and effective and has been used for decades as a treatment for epilepsy. Coconut oil or MCT oil.

You are allowed to have as much cheese, bacon, and butter as you want. You may essentially consume as much fat as you want till you feel satisfied. Eating fat may make you feel satiated.

The Keto diet is effective for people with diabetes. Numerous accounts of people utilizing keto without exercising to lose

50 or even 100 pounds may be found online.

The keto diet is a good option for those with metabolic syndrome, pre-diabetes, or diabetes since it is low in carbohydrates and sugar.

The keto diet might call for a lot of discipline and willpower.

Saying goodbye to all the carbs your body is used to, such as fruit, sweets, bread, and other grains, may be difficult.

It's advised to avoid having a good day on the Keto diet to maximize its effects.

Some people experience the "Keto Flu" when they first begin the diet as their bodies adapt to using fat instead of carbohydrates for fuel.

Despite the Keto diet's lack of restrictions on the variety of food, you will eventually consume less of it. You could have bulletproof coffee for morning (coffee combined with butter and coconut oil), then later on in the day you'll have eggs, some vegetables, and some meat.

It might eventually become monotonous or too constricting.

The What Now: A toolkit for the mind and body, Chapter 4

It was difficult not to incorporate some of the things I discovered via trial and error over the course of the past several years of the trip while putting this book together. This is what I mean when I suggest that everyone who starts anything new (not just a route inside CrossFit) will probably run across some or all of these issues along the way. Here are some things to consider before beginning something new that you may find beneficial to revisit later.

Do you first - You'll have a lot to process in the first weeks and even months, so try not to be distracted by what others are doing. It will be difficult to tell one person apart from another at first just on a few seconds of observation, but as you go forward, you'll eventually uncover certain individuals that you may turn to as role models or for support.

You won't be able to see whether the others around you are doing the routines properly, so focus on the crucial things, like your instructor. It is best to seek advice from your coach rather than copying them.

Since keeping track in your thoughts may be difficult during a set of 100 leaps over a rope or 30 burpees, make it a point to concentrate on counting your repetitions precisely. It's easy to get into complacency while counting and fall back on completing when everyone else finishes. Don't shortchange yourself here; do the job as directed by your coach without taking any short cuts.

It's crucial to take attention of the cues provided while learning a new lift, train your body to really follow them, and remember them for the next time.

Follow your development

Keep track of your results, including your timings, weights for different exercises, and significant achievements like your first double unders or kipping pull-ups. If you need to, bring a notepad with you. I urge you to record the weights and numbers as you begin so that you can keep track of your progress. To be able to recall a previous best lift and surpass it is a really potent workout in and of itself. Knowing how much weight you lifted in the deadlift last month will give you the confidence to record 20 pounds more the following time. Because of this, I've included extra space inside the pages of this book so that you may keep track of these things in one location as you do them.

Know where your metal is: Where you let the equipment fall and where you look when the bar or anything else is above your head are two very important areas to pay attention to. I

With those words:

1) Move out of the way before letting anything fall to the deck.

2) Keep an eye on where the bar, kettlebell, or dumbbell are at all times while doing any overhead exercise, whether it be with a bar, a dumbbell, or both. I

3) For the love of all that is right in the world, maintain your attention on the position of the equipment if the movement compels you to direct your glance on anything else.

4) You'll likely have a large chunk of iron hanging over your head most of the time. You must always be aware of its whereabouts.

Remember, everyone else is working too hard and perspiring too much to pay attention to what anybody else is doing (unless of course it's a high five and congrats on finishing a challenging exercise). "They" are not watching you. You could believe they're keeping an eye on you like hawks, but they're not. Not in the slightest.

Furthermore, if someone is observing you, they are either the coach and doing their job, or they are not the coach and not doing their duty (which is to work hard enough to ignore everything else).

Even with all of this stated, you'll still feel paranoid that Strongman Sven is watching you as you finish your fifth round of 30 burpees, but you'll quickly learn that when you're in the thick of a challenging set of work like that, you don't even hear the music. Therefore, you can be sure that the last thing you'll remember is what the person sitting next to you was doing. Likewise, you can be confident that they won't remember the specifics of what you did either (unless you gave them a celebratory high five at the end, of course).

What you put your attention on expands. Because there is a lot to learn in this area, try to concentrate on the motions and lifts that you find most enjoyable and those you are already naturally skilled at. Others may be really quick runners but struggle to lift heavy weights off the floor. Some folks are great at the dead lift right out of the gate but are sluggish on the rowing machine. Taller people may find it much more efficient to row a fast 800 meters or jump the first leg of a rope climb almost halfway up from the start, whereas shorter people may blow the pants off the taller people in their speed for burpees and their ability to move heavy weights overhead. These ideas are meant to get you thinking about how you might use what you already have to your advantage once you get a sense of what works naturally and what might need extra attention. Of course, there is no real way to categorize what a given person will be good at or need to work harder to improve on.

Giving oneself a mental boost at first is extremely beneficial; focus a LOT of positive thinking on the things you naturally gravitate toward, and as you grow better, concentrate even harder on the remaining tasks. The beautiful thing about CrossFit exercises is that you will always have to do the activities you detest at some time or another, so since you can't avoid them, you may as well be grateful when something you excel at is written across Captain Whiteboard!

Other gym patrons -

Once you get into the swing of things, you'll probably be able to identify folks who are exceptional at everything. Thing. Try to regard these animals as benchmarks to aim towards after you've gained some stability rather than letting it discourage you for falling behind. They understand since they too were new once. Additionally, you'll start to see that fresh individuals will emerge who are in a position comparable to where you were when you first began. Try to make their experience at the gym a good one by introducing yourself when they arrive, cheering them on, assisting them if it seems like they may need a hand, or even completing the exercise with them if you finished it earlier and they are the last ones.

The experience of a new member and the gym as a whole may be greatly impacted by these seemingly little details. We will have more individuals to defend the honor of our CrossFit community, in my opinion, if everyone makes an effort to smile and be generally happy.

You can do this.

Choose a number, memorize it, and use it consistently. Setting the alarm for 5 a.m. and forcing yourself to get out of bed rather than hitting snooze, choosing five days a week to work out in the gym, choosing 20 wall balls before putting the medicine ball down, or powering through an 800 meter row before slowing down are some examples.

Set a limit for yourself and adhere to it. When your muscles and lungs are suffering, let that number ring in your head. The next time the same workout is on your schedule, you'll praise yourself for doing it since you'll know you've done it before and can do it again.

Keep in mind that sustained consistency will lead to progress.

for goodness sake Enjoy yourselves; this isn't a fight to the death. If you fall over your jump rope for the eighth time today, no one is going to run over you and take your shoes. Working alongside individuals that are going through similar problems to you is the greatest because you can look over at your neighbor, encourage them, and grin after it's all said and done knowing that you accomplished more in an hour than 99% of people do in a week.

Be Aware Of Your Body.

Your body will sometimes signal you to do things throughout your CrossFit sessions. This signaling includes a lack of resilience, drive, vitality, and other qualities. You must recognize these warning signals as an athlete before it is too late. These signs may sometimes signify hunger. Sometimes they'll be signs of fatigue. You must always keep oneself in good physical and mental condition. By paying attention to your body, you may prevent training from compromising your performance and, therefore, your outcomes. CrossFit is not a joke, after all. It needs all of your commitment and is physically and mentally demanding. You must totally commit to the training and the art in order to give it your all.

Emotional anguish is often associated with excessive training. Although it is not the root cause, it undoubtedly is a significant contributing component. We already have a lot on our plates between our hectic schedules and other responsibilities, which makes finding time for the things we truly want to accomplish much harder. Anxiety never results in anything positive. You should always strive to improve your work, but not at the expense of your inner tranquility. It's time to change things up if your training routine or approach is making you uneasy. Being uptight is never healthy for your body. No matter how much you try, you just cannot perform at your best. This might result in stiff muscles in your body, which would prevent you from ever getting the most benefit from your activity and increase your chance of injury.

One of the main contributors to issues with anxiety and poor mental health is sleep deprivation. No matter what sport they play, athletes would not be able to perform as effectively as they do without getting the proper amount of sleep. Similar to how your body wants healthy eating to mend itself, it also needs relaxation after an exercise. The time when you sleep is when your body gets the most of that rest. Therefore, you are completely mistaken if you believe that getting up at seven in the morning and staying in bed until two after midnight can provide positive outcomes. While you sleep, your body regenerates. When you remove it from the image, all that's left is a blurry, sleep-deprived version of you. But it goes much beyond just being worn out. You may be surprised to learn that the side effects are far more serious than you would imagine. We haven't even scratched the surface.

The Risks Of Lacking Sleep

I can tell with confidence that I was getting no more than 2 to 3 hours of sleep every night for almost a month. I didn't have to sacrifice either my fitness regimen or my work responsibilities, so I was really content with what I was doing. But my health was what I was inadvertently jeopardizing.

Therefore, my coworkers and I were all anticipating the big day. Everything had been planned out and practiced. Our flights were scheduled. Having even a little margin for mistake was impossible for them since they were perfectionists. Every single issue that we could have predicted was resolved. Then, something unexpected occurred. I became aware that my limbs, notably my arms, were twitching around two days before our journey. Even though I was OK, the waves of sporadic sensations I felt were unlike anything I had ever felt. I put everything behind me and went to sleep that night. I had no sensation in my arms or legs the next morning. They had lost feeling.

I was suffering from anxiety, which had its origins in sleep deprivation. Immediately, I was worried. From either a professional or athletic perspective, I couldn't afford it. I could walk, but not in the way that other people do. I can still see me practically crawling out of bed that morning to get dressed for work. It was just like one of those cliché action movie sequences when the hero is rushing to grab their pistol in the last seconds of their life to rescue the world—or, at the very least, themselves.

I made a call for assistance since I was too sick to drive to work. The problem was that I didn't know why any of it was occurring. My colleagues and I continued to see the situation in a hilarious light throughout the first part of the day. However, we chose to go to the doctor later that day. They conducted several experiments, and the results suggested that they were about to produce something significant. The doctor then told me to sit down and remarked, "You're sleep-deprived." while looking me directly in the eye.

Even while it was reassuring to learn that I wasn't suddenly assaulted by a lethal mutation that took over half of my body, it was terrible to learn how negligent I had been about my health for the previous month or so. Everything made sense when they stated what they said. They didn't have to explain or break things down for me. I knew in my heart of hearts that I just hadn't been getting enough sleep for however long.

That explains why I didn't do as well as normal in the training center during those days. It makes sense why sometimes I struggled to concentrate on the most basic of tasks. The doctor assured me that I had nothing to be concerned about and that all I needed to do was get enough sleep so that once the effects of the tension were gone, my limbs would resume working properly. That also meant that for the next several days or so, I would have to travel with a limp.

In the end, exercise was not an option. I had trouble walking without falling over. I wasn't permitted to put myself under any more pressure. Being unable to workout was a serious setback for me. Additionally, there was the impending presentation that could not be delayed and that I also did not want to cancel. After all, it had been weeks and weeks of nonstop effort that had brought us to that point. We so proceeded with it. The most humiliating thing for me was having to have my traveling companions carry my baggage because whenever I attempted to raise any weight, my hands would simply give out. Being the most physically fit person in the room, I never thought the day would come when I would need help carrying my luggage, which just included a laptop, a charger, some protein bars, and a notepad.

Crossfit Exercises

Cross fit preparation is regarded as a progression of actions meant to improve your molding and quality. Fundamentally, CrossFit preparation focuses mostly on Olympic-style weightlifting. Here are some other schedules you might follow if you wish to attempt this manifestation of preparation. Activities have the ability to practice the most of your body parts, for the most part. It would be simpler for you to get the physique that you have been longing for as a consequence of the comprehensive methods used in this preparation. In the unlikely event that you do encounter this manifestation of preparing, it is crucial for you to be aware of the proportion of cross-fit exercises you may do in the future.

One of the CrossFit exercises that may condition your body is the Indy Routine. Fundamentally, this is a sort of full-body activity and practice that includes body weight squats in addition to pushups. Approximately 20 minutes are allotted for the Indy Routine. This must be completed the next day, and the competitor must confirm that advancement is present. Despite the fact that this program may be completed quickly, it's still one of the most effective fat-burning schedules for CrossFit. However, the Indianapolis Routine is also planned with the intention of adding more muscular bulk to your shoulders and core. In this manner, this concerns your weight loss and body shaping effects.

Additionally regarded as one of the top CrossFit works available is Essy 50. In contrast to the first, this is a rigorous and very demanding kind of exercise. This requires you to do 50 repetitions of 10 different exercises, such as twice unders, burpees, ball hots, back extensions, push presses, lifts, rush tees, kettleball wings, draw ups, and box jumps. Despite the possibility that this kind of routine is really taxing on your body, it will at the moment provide your body the best chance to get more fit and burn more calories, even in only one session. This is why losing weight is undoubtedly one of the benefits of preparing for CrossFit, especially when following this schedule.

Additionally, rough fit preparation is accomplished with the activity known as "Hrusters and Full Ups." This exercise should also be carried out in a monotonous manner. Start the exercise regimen by doing as many push-ups and thrusters as you are able to. You may back off after you are exhausted and have officially completed all the most extreme repetitions. This activity has the effect of smoldering the calories and excess fats present in your stomach region.

L-sit is another among the CrossFit exercises that you may do afterwards. According to the method of this activity, it is great for your stomach and abs. You can, for the most part, shed some of your excess stomach fat by following this schedule. Your legs are straight in front of you while you are supported by your arms in this position.

Twofold Another expansion to your CrossFit routines may be found below. This is essentially a kind of hop rope exercise that will increase your adrenaline rush. This is being done by essentially bouncing over the rope, which ensures that the rope will fall twice before you land on the ground. This routine will compel you to have an increased work capacity. Essentially, this will enhance the activity's calorie-burning effects. Along these lines, this will provide you the chance to effectively become in shape.

a deadlift As another aspect of getting ready for CrossFit, the Lulus Run. This program is regarded as being intense due to the combination of running and deadlifts. This will undoubtedly provide you the chance to eliminate a remarkable amount of belly fat. This will enable you to get more fit in an exceptionally beneficial way. You must do repeated dead lifts throughout this exercise, and you must run for about 1.5 kilometers. This is repeated until you have effectively shown some progress.

Lunges are also among the finest CrossFit exercises. This kind of exercise will improve your whole body's collection of muscles, not just one specific muscle. For example, a ring plunge regimen will provide you more adjustment and quality while simultaneously taking care of the adjustment of rings on the sides of your body. Along these lines, anticipate that this will also cause you to instantly shed too much body fat.

These are some of the activities you may engage in if you want to experience CrossFit preparation in the future. Every activity you support will provide you with extraordinary benefits. This is the reason it would be simple for you to get the physique that you have always yearned for. You will be able to tell that this approach is superior to other projects from health organizations when you experience the effects of the schedules-assisted.

For Runners: Cross Training

A Formula for Effective Running

As they are easier to digest than substantial suppers before a run, those who run longer distances typically utilize protein powder mixes or a dinner substitute powder shortly before making or dashing. Similar to drinking enough water, regular sprinters often include cancer-prevention medications and a high-quality multivitamin supplement to their diets to aid in maintaining energy levels and tissue repair. However, it is evident that food alone, although important, is insufficient. Many sprinters would be shocked to learn that sprinting by itself isn't the most important kind of exercise. The evidence is mounting that wide education may significantly enhance one's running performance. This includes improving one's exhibiting execution to strategy for different sports or training programs in addition to dominating the road or trail. Injury Prevention and Cross Training

Most running competitors who have a wide education cite injury prevention as the main justification for their elective activity. There are many more benefits, but it's important to look at how extensively education might aid in preventing injuries. Veteran sprinters are aware that abuse and mileage are the main causes of the wounds they end up nursing. In any case, it is preferable to explore their origins and determine if there are workable treatments and preventative measures rather than taking them as certainties.

Many athletes fear that taking a break may lead to a decline in wellbeing, which is really not the case. Broadly educating can maintain cardiovascular health, relieve stress from the joints and muscles put under pressure during a run, and increase the strength of the center muscles toward the back and mid-region, which are essential for maintaining proper stance and preventing further injury. Swimming or weightlifting are also excellent ways to relieve joint pain, build resilience and adaptation, promote overall wellbeing, and protect the body from the effects of mileage resulting from running-only exercises.

Cross-training and recovery from injuries

To continue talking about injury for a little while more, general education might be crucial to healing from injury. Some wounds demand constraint from activity if there is any chance of recovery; general education may promote wellbeing and successfully aid the injured tissue in healing. Activities and equipment that are important to running may leave their imprint here. Water running, curved machine cardio (which trains both the upper and lower body using running development without the impact), and inline skating are all excellent alternatives to running.

Increasing Effectiveness

There are a few more benefits to keep in mind. The fact that general education increases strength and production while also increasing speed is perhaps most enticing to sprinters. In general, education allows for more time to be spent exercising, not less, but on activities that will promote cardiovascular health without endangering joints or damaging muscle fibers. The end result is that the person is more physically prepared for a race than would be possible with running-only sessions.

Motivating People

The advantages of widespread education are a different idea. Sprinters run because they like it, but most would admit that there are times when the same routines, streets, and trails may get monotonous. Going for a run while you're tired or furious definitely won't assist the competitor receive the most benefit from the workout. Enhancing running with optional general education practices offers variety, renews motivation, and supports cardiovascular wellbeing in addition to enhancing muscular strength.

Active Restoration

Another important point to remember is the need of a vigorous stretching routine after a run. This is not meant to recommend doing away with rest times entirely after runs. Rest is still necessary to maintaining optimal health, but when done during the first two hours after an activity, a mild dynamic recovery exercise enables the athlete to achieve a far better recovery than simple resting.

Fitness When the season is over

The slower season of the year might be particularly difficult for certain sprinters. The question is whether to run or not to run. Running without rest and recovery may be detrimental, leading to a clearly worse wide presentation the next season rather than a better one. The sluggish season of the year is when better general education may really shine. This doesn't mean that running must be completely stopped, but it may allow for complete rest followed by activities like hockey, ball, swimming, curved training, cycling, weights, yoga, and even hand-to-hand combat. Any one of these (or a combination of a few) may help the body repair the damage from the previous season's misuse while maintaining peak fitness.

The Finding

There is a vast array of generally educational options to look over, and it is important to emphasize once again that they are not intended to replace running as the most important activity but rather to improve and advance it. However, runners should begin to cross rain as soon as possible if they want to avoid injury, recover from an injury effectively, increase their desire to exercise, or increase their speed and efficiency.

Have You Considered The Fat Burning Cross Training Options Yet?

Being a member of the weight loss community puts you head and shoulders over the most popular "copy fat regimens." You may read about them in magazine articles and online features and hear others discussing them. However, have you given it careful thought in order to determine what you want?

Gym put in effort aerobic activity
counting calories

Is Dieting Correct? Naturally, all things considered. It is true. These well-known modalities are effective, but they are also b-o-r-I-n-g. Therefore, it is up to you to think beyond the conventional wisdom about weight loss. Consider delicious meals and enjoyable workouts. How long has it been since you fed or exercised your body to maintain it?

Maybe all the way back to sixth grade? Maybe. OK. The set up is shown below. Your life has gotten much too predictable. You are carrying the extra layers of fat because of this. Since you're worn out, you're insane. It's time to intensify efforts. You should go out on a positive note. also your body.

When preparing your daily dinner, there are several great food types that you should avoid in order to accomplish the fat-consuming task. Consider an antioxidant.

Vegetables
Hearts of artichoke the russet potato
a sweet potato
Veggies and eggplant
Beans
the red beans
kidney bean in red the pinto bean A black bean Fruits
Blueberries
Strawberries
Bilberry
Orange
Grapefruit juice
The Tangerine

How about spices and herbs along with the foods? Cook with them frequently? If you've never cooked using unusual tastes, have you ever eaten them at restaurants or at get-togethers with friends? Then, have courage and look up recipes online and prepare them. Give these fascinating sensations a chance to nourish you and keep you going. You may have the time of your life right now!

As a starting point, consider the following: Chili pepper

Ginger

The Cinna mon Tumer Ic

The movement now. Have you joined a recreation center? No? Great! Here is a thought. Get involved in something that allows you to do what you like. Allow yourself to create your plan. Could it be that you need the recreation center? the exercise equipment? No cost loads? the stairmaster? the population? The coach?

Consider why you need what you require. Do you have any thoughtful information in your head that motivates you to locate the ideal neighborhood recreation facility for you? Perhaps an effort to make the sale? What about this? Consider vacancies in widely educational fields. You are best served by broadly educating yourself since it forces you to consider and make decisions. When a person is thinking and making decisions on their own, their brain creates more synapses.

Recognize that the workout center salesperson has an amount to fill when you are speaking with him. They are selling a software. They speak with authority. The program's cost increases correspond to an improvement in the following check's knock. That is not strange at all. It is a job, and some of those doing it are often quite good at it, therefore they have a right to be highly paid. However, you deserve to have what you want. You may also conduct some research to determine what you want, then sell it to the person working out at the gym.

Pose inquiries to yourself. Find solutions. The list of cross-training exercises is provided below, organized by season:

Winter
Downhill skiing
Cross-country skiing skate on ice
Mountain climbing
The Calisthe Nics
Climbing the Spring Trail
Canoeing
Mountain climbing stairway moving
Cruising Rugby
Rolling about
Water tubing in the summer
Aquatic skiing
Biking
Scuba diving
swimming Climbing a trail
Camping
Surfing Autumn
Leaf rake
Garden harvest
slash wood
Foods may also be frozen. Soccer stairway moving

You can get out of your action box's tiring flow by having fun. Being prepared for your activities is fantastic.

Here is a list of general education activities you may undertake at any time, anywhere.

Yoga

Qi Gong Tai Chi Running Walking

Boxing Swimming

Boxing kicks

Bands, shoot

Dance

the basketball

The Calisthe Nics

By participating in the many cross-training exercises offered, you can make sure that your body gets a decent workout, your brain produces new neuropeptides, your IQ rises, your mood is generally upbeat, and your creativity is boosted and ready to make life richer.

What Makes A Good Breakfast?

In the world of fitness, nutrition is a risky topic. In this book, we'll cover a number of topics, but the main objective is to help you cover your nutritional foundation.

Here are some guidelines for a healthy diet high in fat:

Meets your caloric needs- If you routinely work out at the gym, you'll need to consume more calories than the average person. Lack of caloric intake may initially result in weight loss, but it will ultimately cause a plateau and a decrease in energy.

Proper nutrition mix: Consider your consumption of carbohydrates, proteins, and fats until you find a balance that enhances performance.

Adequate consumption of micronutrients, including essential minerals and vitamins that keep your body functioning and healthy.

Aligned with your goals - Depending on your experience and goals, your diet should take into account what you'd want to accomplish (for example, weight reduction, improved performance, qualifying for a certain CrossFit competition, etc.).

Balanced in a way that encourages longevity- You will find eating to be a terrible experience if your diet does not account for lifestyle factors and chances to "reap the rewards" of your hard work. This makes maintaining long-term health and fitness challenging. A healthy diet allows for occasional treats and cheat meals.

How Do Macronutrients Work?

Macronutrients are the building blocks from which all food for humans is made. A CroFitter has to have a sufficient number of macros to fuel their efforts and recuperate correctly.

The three macronutrients are protein, carbs, and fats. A gram of fat has nine calories, compared to four for a gram of protein, carbohydrates, or both.

The actual building blocks of your diet are proteins. They support the growth of muscle, the regulation of many bodily processes, and hair.

Our efforts are fuelled by carbonates. The body converts carbohydrates into glucose so that we have the energy to do tasks.

Fat regulates a number of hormonal processes in our bodies and maintains the health of our nervous system.

All machines are not created evenly, even if their caloric value never varies. Because they include omega-3 fatty acids, monounsaturated and polyunsaturated fats are regarded as the "healthy fats," whereas saturated fats are seen differently. They are both fat, which means they both have 9 calories per grain, in any case.

How Do Micronutrients Work?

Micronutrients are substances like vitamins and minerals that a healthy body need to operate properly. They are necessary for things like disease prevention, growth, and wellbeing.

Examples include iron, vitamin A, dodine, and zinc. For instance, a ron deficiency might hinder cognitive and motor development.

You can get the most micronutrients by consuming a diet high in lean meats, vegetables, and fruits.

Foods to avoid before an exercise include raw vegetables.

Avoid eating any vegetables that might give you stomach discomfort before you begin your exercise. This includes vegetables like lettuce, cabbage, and broccoli that are often consumed raw. They are nutritious and high in fiber, however they are not advised for pre-workout meals.

High-Ugah Carb

High-glycemic carbohydrates will obviously spike your blood sugar and impede you from losing weight and building muscle. Avoid high-sugar carbohydrates like bread, potatoes, and white rice, even if you get them from natural sources. You still need carbohydrates, but they should come from whole grains.

Another off-limits item in the world of CrossFit is fried food. And let's face it, you don't need a lengthy explanation of why fried foods are bad for your health. The simplest explanation is that fried foods lack nourishment and are high in trans fats, which deplete energy levels. Instead of feeling energized, you'll feel lethargic, making it impossible for you to complete your workday.

Alcohol

Any alcohol is a high-calorie beverage, so if you're trying to lose weight, you should stay away from it. This is why you should avoid it as much as possible while following the CrFit diet plan. You won't get any lower than alcohol.

Fried foods and processed foods fall under the same category. Crackers, granola bars, and pastries are strictly forbidden. Processed foods that are high in sugar may lengthen your wait time and make your Croissant work very impossible to complete.

flavor-infused yogurt

This is certainly the most alluring choice. Although yogurt is a terrific snack, flavoring it won't help you build muscle. Despite the protein, flavoring yoghurt is something you should stay away from.

The reason is straightforward: Flavored yogurt is high in sugar and sodium. You'll feel exhausted and bruised afterward.

Worst Food for Children

You're working out like a beast, but if you fill up on these foods, you're not doing yourself any favors. Avoid them just like you would avoid the reputation of being "skinny fat"!

1. Raw vegetables before exercise

Avoid eating lettuce, cabbage, and broccoli before working out, advises Hayim. The Mayo Clinic claims that these foods are common causes of stomach pain. While they may be healthy and high in fiber, they might cause discomfort during an exercise, particularly during an intensive one like CrossFit. Additionally, you don't want to be that uncomfortable, gassy person in class, do you? So not sexy.

2.High-Fructose Carbohydrates

Avoid high-sugar carbohydrates, even if they come from a natural source, advises Smiley. "White rice, potatoes, and bread are off-limits because they are abnormally high in the glycemic index, which will spike your insulin levels and then cause them to drop, sending you spiraling through hunger alley looking for a sweet treat."

But when it comes to carbohydrates, don't go cold turkey. "Whole grains are complex carbohydrates, meaning they breakdown slowly in your body, allowing your body to absorb several nutrients. After that intense 25-minute AMRAP CrossFit session, carbohydrates are digested and absorbed as glycogen, which will replenish depleted muscle tissue.

The proper carbohydrate sources will provide CrossFit competitors the ongoing energy and endurance they need to complete every repetition they are due. Portion control carbs and often consume whole grains, fruits, and vegetable-based sources of carbohydrates including quinoa, farro, sweet potatoes, beets, and more.

3. Frozen Foods

Let's face it, you don't need a long explanation of why these oily, crispy globs are unhealthy. So here is a brief one: CrossFit is a demanding activity that requires the best nutrition to fuel it. Fried foods deplete your energy levels and make you lethargic since they are nutritionally unhealthy and rich in unhealthy saturated and trans fats. And lest we forget, there are foods that speed up the aging process as well. Yes, we didn't believe you were interested in it either, to be honest.

4. Boulder cubes

A little post-workout rough? Hold on. These may be wonderful for creating tasty soups, but they are loaded with a significant amount of salt, warns Hayim. "You need to concentrate on replacing your daily fluid losses while your body is healing. While a little amount of salt in the diet might be beneficial for athletes, the salt in bouillon can cause dehydration, which can eventually affect your muscles' ability to contract during a workout.

5.Alcohol

Okay, you know not to drink frozen beverages while doing CrossFit training, but even one or two glasses of wine may ruin your exercise routine, according to William. "Nothing will slow you down quite like alcohol, with lasting negative effects on CrossFit training and performance." "Alcohol is just empty calories since it has no nutritional value. Additionally, it has been shown to disregard recovery and disrupt sleep, two crucial elements in any training program!" Check out what happens to your body when you quit drinking alcohol for inspiration to move away from alcohol temporarily.

6. Prepared food

Granola bars, restaurants, and even crackers should all have "You're Fired" Donald Trump statues. when it comes to your poor performance. Foods that have been processed can include unhealthy and unnatural substances. The sugar will lengthen your waistline, making those pull-ups, push-ups, and handstand push-ups much harder, according to William. And really, who needs that? "Also, these processed treatments do not provide the nutrient density that whole foods deliver, leaving your body short of necessary nutrients to aid in recovery," the article continues. Simply avoid them. Your body will appreciate you.

7. Bagels

We are aware of how alluring a bagel with an indulgent schmear of cream cheese may be as a handy on-the-go food.Unfortunately, most athletes feel drained rather than energized after eating bagels because of their high-carb, high-glycemic index. Do you feel you should take a pre-workout supplement to boost your energy?Most recent nutrition research is dispelling the age-old idea that carbo-loading before exercise is beneficial.

8. At the movies, popcorn

Making a Friday night move to avoid the bars and clubs before a big Thanksgiving day? Go ahead and order it, but be sure to stay away from the popcorn. While movie theater popcorn seems to be the least dangerous option available at the concession stand, it is loaded with salt and saturated fat from the butt. Hayim warns that partaking in this activity the night before your workday may result in bleeding and early muscle fatigue. You may be able to stop belly fat quickly, but your exercise performance will still suffer.

9.Hamburgers

You're exerting so much effort to cover your abdomen; why ruin it with a greasy calorie bomb?Loading up on fatty, hefty items like hamburgers or fries is a kind of diet sabotage. Workouts become more difficult when there is an abundance of harmful fats that are difficult to digest. "Healthy fats, on the other hand, provide energy and help rather than obstruct the digestive system," the author writes. Choose these meals for x-pack abs since they are the greatest for those killer abs.

No. 10 Flavored Yogurt

It's challenging yet instructive. Flavored yogurt doesn't aid in recovery or muscle development, asserts Hayim. It has two times less protein than Greek yogurt and is laden with salt and sugar, all of which make you feel exhausted and bloated. If you're in the mood for something sweeter, try combining plain, unsweetened Greek yogurt with sliced banana, chia seeds, and honey for a healthy but indulgent treat.

Cross-Training With A Paleo Diet

The goal of diet and exercise is to work together to promote wellbeing and strength. Coach Greg Glassman developed the concept of cross training over the course of several years. There are several fitness establishments that provide it as a business structure, but you may also do it on your own. It often contains lots of constantly changing severe concentration techniques. Due to the fact that the timetables are based on regular advances, it is a utilitarian sort of activity. For instance, taking care of something on a high rack could need comparable muscles and development as a Cross Training exercise. Cross training and other extreme concentration techniques have shown to be effective fat burners. It is wiser to do a unique workout vigorously for a little period of time than to repeat the same activity repeatedly for a very long time. When you do an intense concentration workout to stimulate your digestion, your body continues to consume fat even after the exercise is over. More fat is being consumed faster than anticipated. Walking quickly and enthusiastically burns more calories than slow, leisurely walking over long distances. The typical cross-training workout takes somewhere between two and thirty minutes to complete. Broad education might be a relaxed approach to health and recovery or an intense one for muscle fanatics.

Visit CrossFit.com if you're interested in learning more about cross training or trying out some of the exercises. Generally speaking, depending on your goals, it is advised to choose between the Paleo diet and the Zone weight-control program. The vast majority of Cross mentors also adhere to a Paleo diet. People with a general education are interested in gaining as much energy from their meals as is logically possible. They do this by including more healthy fats into their diets, such as nuts and olives. The Paleo diet pairs well with this. Instead of higher glycemic food sources like most carbohydrates, they increase the variety of low glycemic food choices. Due to the fact that Paleo really allows you to consume a lot of food, general education works quite well with it. You may have a variety of smaller meals throughout the day. Cross Training and Paleo both see food as bodily fuel.

Positive results may be obtained with either the Paleo diet or Cross preparation. The finest results may be obtained in the shortest amount of time by pursuing both as a way of life. Paleo and cross training ought to be doable on your own terms.

Chapter 3: Foods That Will Ruin Your Life and Paleo Fanatics The annoying thing about any devotee is that, regardless of how terrible they are right now, in a month they will be a fan of something else and still be awful.

If you've read widely educational books, you probably already know that I often discuss a modified Paleo diet. When I say "adjusted," I mean that I don't exactly follow every single one of the rules established by the very sane Paleo folks organization. If you must, it means you approve of me. A substantial number of us choose Paleo in order to feel healthier and obtain a more toned figure. It has been shown that you can achieve this goal while adhering to the Paleo diet around 80% of the time. Let's be honest: if we have unreasonable expectations of ourselves, we won't ever stick to any eating plans. A good eating regimen must be flexible enough to fit into a life that is actually ordinary. Do these Paleo enthusiasts isolate themselves from others? Do they not operate a car? I'm happy to inform that the Paleo diet may help you lose weight and improve your health without requiring you to be a diehard follower.

The information on the Paleo period intrigues me. I acknowledge that a lot of it is true. In any event, there are many theories because, let's face it, it was a long time ago. So I don't really need the mountain guy stuff. Results, though, are crucial. I said before that there are two ways to adhere to the Paleo diet. You may either adhere to it strictly or more often than not. The two of them also have a job. You must adhere to it completely if you are having immune system problems. The majority of the time, Paleo will work out well for you if all you're trying to do is reduce your muscle to fat ratio and feel considerably better. Therefore, the demands for me are not coming from prehistoric men. The fact that Paleo appears reasonable and helps a lot of people become fitter and feel better really speaks to me. Why does Paleo accomplish this? I'll try to put it simply: I'm a truly negatively vulnerable kind of person. I'm not a professional or researcher, but throughout the years, I've gained a lot of valuable experience with hypersensitivity.

It is a truth. Grain, dairy, and other proteins are avoided by many people's systems. The body's reaction to these things it doesn't like is hypersensitivity. The majority of them are solid proteins. The body's effort to protect itself against proteins it doesn't trust results in the adverse effects. In conclusion, when your body is exposed to something it doesn't like, it is essentially telling you: "There's this protein I don't know about." I shall make an effort to eliminate whatever parasite or bacterium is seeking to harm me. Now, although it is undoubtedly a clever way to say it, the hypersensitive response is essentially that (really). Therefore, the body makes an effort to eliminate what it believes to be a parasite, microbe, or other threatening entity. To get rid of it, it releases substantial amounts of synthetic compounds. These include substances like cortisol, histamine, and others. Your security plan suggests a commercial setting. As a result, the situation is one of annoyance from the beginning. There will be an irritant. Your sinus passages will be irritated and expanded if it's dust in your nose. In the worst-case scenario, your body would be attacking itself. The core concept of immune system diseases is that the body is harming itself.

Although it is a bothersome immune system disorder, hay fever is really harmless. If this situation develops in a different way, you might have diabetes or other serious, harmful health problems. In reality, comparable types of proteins cause excessive sensitivity in the great majority of people with food hypersensitivities. Additionally, consider what they are. Vegetables, dairy, and grains are often combined. Indeed, it is a common problem for some sensitive people. However, even if you are not allergic to anything that you are aware of, your body nonetheless could react to these proteins. Many individuals continue to consume foods that, at best, make their lives unpleasant and costly while also slowly killing them. You may have been consuming food types that irritate your body ever since you were a child. I speak honestly because I am aware of it. The good news is that once these irritants are eliminated, the inflammation subsides and you feel better.

That's not all, however. It has often been shown that grains, carbohydrates, and sweets also contribute to our weight gain. Likewise, food additives are. Significant illnesses like heart ailments and unexpected cerebral problems like dementia have been linked to additives. So, the aspect about Paleo that I adore is this.

You'll continue to read articles on wheat and other grains and their links to diabetes and other diseases. Paleo is really the best eating plan for the majority of us and will provide amazing results. Therefore, whether or not there is a mountain man living in the cavern, this eating plan works and produces results. The key thing is that this is the eating plan we should be following if we want to look amazing and feel fantastic, whether you call it the Paleo diet or the Caveman diet. Paleo with a different name.

How Many Blocks Do You Need

Your sex, body type, and level of activity determine how many blocks you need each day.

The average-sized woman needs 11 blocks daily of each macronutrient category—carbohydrate, protein, and fat—while the average-sized male needs 14 blocks. Using the meal chart provided by CrossFit, you may count your blocks. You may also use the Body Fat Calculator on the Zon for a more accurate estimate. Once you are aware of your block count, you should only split your blocks into meals and snacks to ensure a balance of carbs, protein, and fat. An average-sized woman requires 3 blocks of each macronutrient during meals as opposed to an average-sized male who requires 4 blocks per macronutrient. Additional 1-2 blocks of each macronutrient are consumed as snacks.

Block amples

For a three-block breakfast, you would need three portions of protein, carbs, and fat. Using a block chart, you can see that one block of carbohydrates equals one-third of a cup of cooked oats. You might consume one cup of cooked oatmeal to get three blocks. Similar to that, 1/4 cup of cheddar counts as one proton block. Eat a 3/4 cup of cottage cheese to get three blocks. Finally, three almonds equal one fat block. Therefore, consuming 9 almonds would result in 3 blocks.

Food Weighing and Measuring

You are permitted to estimate the serving sizes of foods and good carbs using the hand-eye method in accordance with the CrossFit-recommended Zone Diet guidelines. That entails choosing proteins, such as meat, that are around the size and thickness of the palm of your hand (3-4 cooked ounces), then making about two-thirds of your plate out of vegetables, and a small amount of fruit. To improve your ability to estimate food quantities, you must weigh and measure your dishes for at least one week.

www.ingramcontent.com/pod-product-compliance
Lightning Source LLC
Chambersburg PA
CBHW070033040426
42333CB00040B/1594